GAPS Diet

Heal Intestinal Issues And Prevent Autoimmune Diseases (Leaky Gut, Gastrointestinal Problems, Gut Health, Reduce Inflammation)

Sherry S. Williams

GAPS Diet: Heal Intestinal Issues And Prevent Autoimmune Diseases (Leaky Gut, Gastrointestinal Problems, Gut Health, Reduce Inflammation)

Table of Contents

1 - What the GAPS Diet is All About..........................1
    For Your Gut's Sake..........................1
    Health Benefits Abound..........................2

2 - GAPS Guidelines..........................3

3 - The GAPS Introduction Diet..........................6

4 - First Stage..........................7
    Consume meat/fish stock that you make yourself..........................7
    Tips:..........................8
    Consume soups prepared with your homemade meat and fish stocks..........................9
    Start eating fermented foods that can be vegetable-based or dairy-based..........................9
    Take ginger tea (enriched with a bit of honey) before and after meals..........................10

5 - Second Stage..........................11
    Carry on with the foods introduced in the first stage of the Introduction Diet..........................11
    Add egg yolks (go for raw and organic) to your diet..........................11
    Consume casseroles and stews made with vegetables and meats..........................12
    Start consuming kefir and yogurt (homemade)..........................12
    Start eating fermented fish..........................12
    Begin using ghee in your meals..........................13

6 - Third Stage..........................14
    Incorporate ripe avocado to your soups..........................14
    Have some pancakes..........................14
    Consume scrambled eggs cooked with lots of ghee, duck fat, or goose fat..........................14
    Eat fermented vegetables..........................15

7 - Fourth Stage..........................16
    Continue..........................16
    Gradually eat grilled and roasted meats (avoid any fried or barbecued options for now)..........................16
    Start using olive oil (make sure it is cold pressed)..........................16
    Begin enjoying freshly pressed vegetable juices..........................17
    Consider eating breads baked with nut flours (almond flour is an excellent choice)..........................17

8 - Fifth Stage..........................18
    Given that your gut and body have been able to tolerate all the foods introduced from the first to the fourth stage..........................18
    Start eating raw vegetables..........................18

Start adding fruit juice to your diet..19

9 - Sixth Stage...20
Granting that your body has no problems with all of the foods introduced from the first stage down to the fifth stage............20
Slowly increase the amount of baked goods and sweet treats in your diet..20

10 - List of Foods to Eat..21

11 - List of Foods to Avoid......................................32

12 - Breakfast..42
Nutty Coconut Granola..42
Cheddar Nettle Omelet..43
Cinnapple Pancakes...45
Breakfast Cookies...46
Crumbly Almond Blueberry Breakfast Muffins.........48
Cream Cheese & Carrot Morning Cupcakes..............50

13 - Lunch...53
Tarragon & Mustard Chicken..................................53
Savory Onion Soup...55
Mustard & Leek Carrot Soup...................................57
Steak with Wild Mushroom Sauce...........................59
Beef & Root Veggies Stew..61
Dill-Onion Chicken Roast.......................................63
Lemon Sole...65

14 - Dinner..67
Coconut Lemongrass Chicken Soup.........................67
Veggie Seafood Stew...69
Easy Burger Salads...72
Red Wine Bison Stew..74
Walnut Beet Salad...76
Smokin' Salmon Roe...78
Tasty Rosemary Steak...79

15 - Condiments...81
Hot Garlic Kraut...81
Easy Green Chile Salsa..82
GAPS-Friendly Pepperoncini...................................83
No-Fuss Sauerkraut..85
Fennel & Cucumber Pickles.....................................86

16 - Spreads..88
Bacon-Shallot Potted Cheddar................................88
Homemade Avocado Oil Mayo.................................89
Honey Whiskey Marmalade.....................................90
Easy Sage Pate...92
Delish Dill Mayo...94

17 - Beverages..96
Kombucha Cranberry Slushy...................................96

Nourishing Ginger Tea..96
Gut-Friendly Soda...98
Fermented Green Tea..99
Lime Apple Tonic...100
Heartwarming Mulled Wine...101
Invigorating Water Kefir..102

18 - Snacks And Treats..105

Blood Orange & Coconut Jelly-Mousse....................................105
Nutty Strawberry Bowl with Yogurt......................................108
Creamy Coconut Ice Cream..110
Lemon-Thyme Toasted Almonds..111
Roasted Cabbage Wedges...112
Lentil Chili Snack..113
Minty Strawberry Sorbet..115
Honeyed Berry Mix..116

19 - Baked Goods..118

Blueberry Banana Pudding...118
Easy Apple Crumble...120
Carrot Cupcakes...121
Tasty Pumpkin Bread..124
Delicious Banana Bread...125

Thank You..127

Disclaimer..128

1 - What the GAPS Diet is All About

The GAPS Diet is one that helps you forego foods that your body finds difficult to digest and that damage your gut flora, recommending instead that you consume foods that have high nutrient value and that allow your intestinal lining the opportunity to get healed and sealed.

For Your Gut's Sake

When you really think about it, the GAPS Diet allows you to enjoy your meals while feeding your body with foods that help in:

- Repairing your intestinal wall/addressing a problem with a leaky gut

- Rebalancing the good bacteria and bad bacteria numbers in your gut

- Preventing bad bacteria from dominating your gut environment and overloading it with toxins

- Protecting you from various autoimmune diseases caused by the flooding of gut toxins in your bloodstream

- Letting your gut as well as your body rest and restore themselves while you eat foods that can be easily digested

Health Benefits Abound

By following the GAPS Diet plan, you reap the benefits of having a healthy gut:

- Reduced sensitivity to certain foods

- Resolved inflammatory bowel issues

- Improved digestion of lactose

- Elimination of candida

- Improved detoxification in your body

- Enhanced immunity, neurological function, and autism

- Reversed diabetes (type II) condition

- Reduced feelings of anxiety and depression

2 - GAPS Guidelines

At the heart of the GAPS Diet plan are the fermented foods, which include yogurt, sour cream, fermented vegetables, and fermented beverages (water kefir, kombucha, and kvass).

During your first weeks on the GAPS diet, you might find these types of foods difficult to tolerate, so that it would be a good idea to avoid eating them temporarily. As you gradually introduce fermented foods into your diet, make sure to observe how your body reacts and note any negative reactions.

Accompanying each of your meals with once cup of meat stock or bone broth is recommended on the GAPS diet. In the early days or weeks, your digestive system may have trouble digesting fats, which is why you would be better off taking only two to three tablespoons of meat stock or bone broth until your body has healed.

The GAPS diet encourages the consumption of raw, cooked, or fermented vegetables along with fish and meat. This is to promote pH balance in your body: Fish and meat are converted to acids in your body, and the vegetables will help neutralize these acids with their strong alkalizing property.

To keep fruits from hampering your digestion when eating meats, it would be best to consume fruit before or after meals (with the exception of avocado).

If your body and your gut can tolerate it, consider the GAPS diet recommendation to add lots of natural fats to each of your meals. Good fat choices include olive oil (cold pressed), coconut oil, and animal fats such as butter (raw), ghee (raw), lard, duck fat, lamb fat, and tallow.

Keep in mind that a large chunk of your diet when following the GAPS diet plan should comprise of vegetables (fermented, cooked or raw), fermented foods, fish, shellfish, farm-fresh eggs (organic is best), fresh meats (grass fed or hormone-free is preferred), and animal fats.

Avoid eating too much baked goods, especially those made with fruit and nut flours; it is best to eat them in moderate amounts, as overindulgence can interfere with your body's healing process. In case you suffer from a yeast infection, you might consider temporarily foregoing honey, fruits and nuts.

As animals have a built-in detoxification system that can neutralize hormones or antibiotics (a small part) used on them, you may be better off purchasing local/organic and pesticide-free vegetables and fruits instead of fresh (organic) or frozen meats.

Remember to eliminate all packaged processed foods from your diet, which can negatively impact your digestive and healing processes. Avoid eating all forms of refined carbohydrates as well as all foods that are made with chemicals like preservatives and artificial colorants.

3 - The GAPS Introduction Diet

The GAPS Introduction Diet (involving six stages) is recommended for you if you are suffering from diarrhea, constipation, bloating, abdominal pain, and other serious digestive symptoms. Going on the Introduction Diet will help you transition to the Full GAPS Diet, as the former helps decrease your symptoms fast as well as initiate your digestive system's healing process.

4 - First Stage

Consume meat/fish stock that you make yourself

Stocks made from meat and fish supply your body with the building blocks it needs to quickly regenerate cells in your gut lining. They are also effective in soothing any part of your gut that is affected with inflammation. This is the reason homemade meat/fish stocks are able to support good digestion.

To prepare your meat or fish stock at home, fill a large pan with water and then the bones and joints. Add the meats as well as unprocessed salt (1 teaspoon) and roughly crushed black peppercorns (1 teaspoon), then allow the mixture to come to a boil.

Reduce heat, cover the pan, and simmer for about three hours. Once done, remove the meats and bones, and then strain the stock to separate the peppercorns and small bones. Make sure to reserve all soft meat parts attached to the bones; you can use them later in making homemade soups.

Tips:

Avoid using stock granules, bouillon cubes, or other forms of commercially made soups. These were made using extensive processing and contain plenty of gut-harming ingredients. You might consider getting started with chicken stock, which is known to be especially gently on the tummy.

Make sure to use bones, joints, a whole chicken, a whole pigeon, meat pieces that are attached to the bone, chicken giblets, pheasants, duck, goose, or other cheap meats. This ensures that you will be able to make good quality meat stock.

Remember that bones and joints are what you are truly after – the healing substances from a good meat stock come from them, not from the meat parts. It would be a good idea to have the tubular bones cut in half by the butcher; this way, you can easily extract the bone marrow once the bones (bang on a clean wooden board while still warm) are cooked.

Consume the bone marrow and gelatinous soft tissues surrounding the bones after each meal. They are rich in healing substances that your gut lining as well as immune system need to recover.

You can refrigerate or freeze your homemade meat and fish stocks for up to one week.

Consume soups prepared with your homemade meat and fish stocks

Add fermented foods to each bowl of soup you consume. You can consume these homemade soups with soft bone tissues and meat (boiled) all through the day.

Start eating fermented foods that can be vegetable-based or dairy-based.

You can avoid experiencing reactions by simply making sure to eat fermented foods at this stage in a gradual manner. Begin by eating just one to two teaspoons of fermented foods for two to five days. Increase your intake to three to four teaspoons for another two to five days, after which you can then add several teaspoons to each bowl of meat stock and soup that you eat.

When adding fermented foods, see to it that your meat/fish stock or soup is not that hot – extreme heat can easily destroy any beneficial bacteria present in the added fermented foods.

Take ginger tea (enriched with a bit of honey) before and after meals.

You can easily prepare ginger tea by grating a fresh piece of ginger root. Take one teaspoon of the grated ginger and place in a teapot. Add enough boiling water to submerge the ginger, then cover the teapot and let the ginger sit for about three to five minutes. Strain through a fine-mesh sieve before pouring into a mug. Stir in one teaspoon of honey, sip and enjoy.

5 - Second Stage

Carry on with the foods introduced in the first stage of the Introduction Diet.

Keep on consuming meat stocks, fish stocks, soups from said stocks, fermented foods, and ginger tea.

Add egg yolks (go for raw and organic) to your diet

You can add the raw egg yolks to each cup of meat/fish stock you drink and each bowl of homemade soup you consume. You can begin by adding one egg yolk per day, then slowly increase the number of egg yolks until you are consuming one egg yolk with every stock cup or soup bowl.

If you find that you can easily tolerate egg yolks, you may step it up by adding soft-boiled eggs to your soups – the egg whites should be cooked but the egg yolks should still be runny. To ease your mind with regard to issues with egg allergies, consider performing an egg sensitivity test first.

Know that you do not have to restrict yourself in terms of the quantity of egg yolks you can consume in a day. Egg yolks are quickly absorbed by your body, do not require your digestive system to work so much, and can supply your body the nutrients it needs.

Consume casseroles and stews made with vegetables and meats

Just remember to stay away from spices at this point in the Introduction Diet. You can prepare your stews with fresh herbs and unprocessed salt, and make sure they contain high amounts of fat. Your body will recover at a faster rate if your meals contain higher amounts of fresh animal fats. Don't forget to add fermented foods to each serving of casserole or stew.

Start consuming kefir and yogurt (homemade)

You can also increase your intake of the juices from fermented foods like sauerkraut and other fermented veggies at this stage of the Introduction Diet.

Start eating fermented fish

Work on eating one piece daily, then gradually increasing the amount.

Begin using ghee in your meals

A good way to start is by consuming one teaspoon daily before gradually increasing the amount.

6 - Third Stage

Continue eating all the foods introduced in the first and second stages of the Introduction Diet

Incorporate ripe avocado to your soups

Start by adding one to three teaspoons of mashed avocado to your meals, and then gradually increase the number of teaspoons or tablespoons.

Have some pancakes

Begin by consuming including one pancake daily in your diet, then slowly increase the number of pancakes. To get you started, you can quickly whip up pancakes by using no more than three ingredients. Combine fresh zucchini (peeled, deseeded and spiralized) with eggs and organic almond butter; use ghee/duck fat/goose fat to fry; and serve immediately.

Consume scrambled eggs cooked with lots of ghee, duck fat, or goose fat

You can serve these scrambled eggs with cooked vegetables and ripe avocado. To help boost your digestive system as well as your immune system, try low-heat cooking white onion slices in three tablespoons of melted ghee for about twenty to thirty minutes.

Eat fermented vegetables

You have been drinking their juices during the second stage of the Introduction Diet. Now is the time for you to actually eat them. A good way to start is by eating one to two tablespoons of sauerkraut and other fermented vegetables with each meal, then slowly increasing their quantities.

7 - Fourth Stage

Continue

Continue eating all the foods you have consumed during the first, second, and third stages of the Introduction Diet

Gradually eat grilled and roasted meats (avoid any fried or barbecued options for now).

Make sure to avoid eating any overly browned or burnt bits of meat. Consume your grilled/roasted meat with sauerkraut/other fermented veggies as well as cooked vegetables.

Start using olive oil (make sure it is cold pressed)

You can add about two to three drops of olive oil to your every meal and then slowly work your way up to adding one to two tablespoons to every meal.

Begin enjoying freshly pressed vegetable juices.

You can start by taking a couple of tablespoons of freshly made, well-filtered, clear carrot juice. You can slowly drink the carrot juice as is, or mix it with a dollop of homemade yogurt or five to six tablespoons of warm water.

Once you have worked your way up to drinking one whole cup of clear carrot juice, you can try adding it to other vegetable juices (good choices include fresh mint leaves, lettuce, and celery). Make sure to consume vegetable juices when your stomach is empty, such as the moment you wake up in the morning or a few hours after lunch.

Consider eating breads baked with nut flours (almond flour is an excellent choice)

You may start baking your GAPS-friendly bread with just four ingredients. Combine eggs and nut flour with spiralized winter squash, salt, and butter/ghee. Eat one slice per day, then gradually increase the quantity.

8 - Fifth Stage

Given that your gut and body have been able to tolerate all the foods introduced from the first to the fourth stage.

You can consider adding apple puree (cooked apple) to your meals. Start by peeling and coring ripe apples. Soften the apples by stewing in a little water, add ghee, duck fat, or goose fat, and mash thoroughly. Eat just one to two teaspoons per day to check if you get any reaction. Otherwise, continue eating the apple puree and gradually increase the number of teaspoons or tablespoons.

Start eating raw vegetables

You can add the softer parts of raw lettuce and cucumber (peeled) to your meals. Just make sure to check your stool for any reaction. It would be best to begin introducing raw veggies at this point in small amounts, then gradually increase the amount if your body is able to tolerate them.

Once your body has gotten used to lettuce and cucumber, you can begin adding raw tomatoes, cabbages, carrots, and onions.

Start adding fruit juice to your diet

Try mango juice, apple juice, and pineapple juice. At this point, it would be best to avoid having any juice made with citrus fruits.

9 - Sixth Stage

Granting that your body has no problems with all of the foods introduced from the first stage down to the fifth stage

You may add raw (peeled) apple at this point. You may also start eating raw fruit during this stage in the Introduction Diet. Adding more honey to your foods should be tolerated by your body at this point.

Slowly increase the amount of baked goods and sweet treats in your diet

Make sure to use only dried fruit as your natural sweetener.

10 - List of Foods to Eat

- Almonds

- Almond oil

- Almond butter

- Apples

- Fresh/dried apricots

- French artichoke

- Asiago cheese

- Asparagus

- Eggplant (aborigine)

- Avocados

- Avocado oil

- Ripe bananas (skin w/ brown spots)

- Dried white/navy beans

- String beans

- Lima beans

- Fresh/frozen beef

- Beets/beetroot

- All kinds of berries

- Ground red pepper, black pepper, and white pepper

- Red, black, and white peppercorns

- Radish (black)

- Cheese, blue

- Bok Choy

- Nuts, Brazil

- Cheese, brick

- Cheese, brie

- Broccoli

- Brussels sprouts

- Grass-fed butter

- Cabbage

- Cheese, Camembert

- Fish, canned (water-/oil-packed)

- Capers

- Carrots

- Fresh cashew nuts

- Cauliflower

- Pepper, cayenne

- Celery

- Celery root

- Cheese, cheddar

- Cherimoya (sharifa/custard apple)

- Cherries

- Fresh/frozen chicken

- Cinnamon

- Citric acid

- Fresh/dried coconut (shredded & additive-free)

- Coconut milk

- Virgin coconut oil

- Freshly made coffee (weak, not instant)

- Greens, collard

- Cheese, Colby

- Zucchini (courgette)

- Fresh/dried coriander

- Cucumber

- Fresh/dried dates (additive-free, syrup-free)

- Fresh/dried dill

- Fresh/frozen duck

- Cheese, Edam

- Aubergine (eggplant)

- Fresh eggs

- Filberts

- Fresh/frozen/canned fish

- Fresh/frozen game

- Garlic

- Homemade ghee

- Gin (on occasions)

- Fresh ginger root

- Fresh/frozen goose

- Cheese, gorgonzola

- Cheese, Gouda

- Grapefruit

- Grapes

- Beans, haricot

- Cheese, Havarti

- Hazelnuts

- Teas, herbal

- Fresh/dried herbs (additive-free)

- Natural honey

- Juices from permitted vegetables & fruits (freshly

pressed)

- Kale

- Kiwi

- Kumquats

- Fresh/frozen lamb

- Lemons

- Lentils

- All kinds of lettuce

- Fresh/dried lima beans

- Cheese, Limburger

- Limes

- Mangoes

- Fresh/frozen meat

- Melons

- Cheese, Monterey Jack

- Cheese, Muenster

- Mushrooms

- Mustard seeds

- Nectarines

- Almond meal

- Almond flour

- Nutmeg

- All kinds of nuts (freshly shelled, not salted/coated/pre-roasted)

- Cold-pressed olive oil (virgin)

- Olives (sugar-free)

- Onions

- Oranges

- Papayas

- Cheese, Parmesan

- Parsley

- Peaches

- Additive-free peanut butter

- Fresh/roasted peanuts (with intact shells)

- Pears

- Fresh green peas

- Dried split peas

- Pecans

- Red peppers

- Yellow peppers

- Green peppers

- Orange peppers

- Fresh/frozen pheasant

- Sugar-free pickles

- Fresh/frozen pigeon

- Fresh pineapples

- Fresh/frozen pork

- Cheese, Port du Salut

- Fresh/frozen poultry

- Dried prunes (additive-free)

- Canned prunes (in own juice)

- Pumpkin

- Fresh/frozen quail

- Raisins

- Rhubarb

- Cheese, Roquefort

- Cheese, Romano

- Satsumas

- Scotch (on occasions)

- Fresh/dried seaweed – upon completion of GAPS Introduction Diet

- Fresh/frozen shellfish

- Pure & single spices (additive-free)

- Spinach

- Summer squash

- Winter squash

- Cheese, Stilton

- String beans

- Swedes

- Cheese, Swiss

- Tangerines

- Freshly made tea (weak, not instant)

- Pure tomato puree (additive-free)

- Tomato juice (additive-free)

- Tomatoes

- Fresh/frozen turkey

- Turnips

- Ugli fruit

- Cheese, cottage (uncreamed/dry curd)

- White/cider vinegar (allergen-free)

- Vodka (on rare occasions)

- Walnuts

- Watercress

- Dry red wine

- Dry white wine

- Homemade yogurt

11 - List of Foods to Avoid

- Acesulphame

- Milk, acidophilus

- Agar-agar

- Agave syrup

- Algae

- Aloe Vera

- Amaranth

- Commercial apple juice

- Arrowroot

- Aspartame

- Astralagus

- Beans prepared by baking

- Baker's yeast

- Raising agents, including baking powder

- Balsamic vinegar

- Barley
- Bean sprouts
- Bean flour
- Bee pollen
- Beer
- Okra (bhindi)
- Sodium bicarbonate
- Bitter gourd
- Beans, black eye
- Bologna
- Bouillon granules/cubes
- Brandy
- Buckwheat flour
- Bulgur
- Root, Burdock
- Beans, butter

- Buttermilk

- Beans, cannellini

- Canned vegetables

- Canned fruits

- Carob

- Carrageenan

- Cellulose gum

- All kinds of breakfast cereal

- Processed cheeses

- Processed cheese spreads

- Chestnuts

- Chestnut flour

- Cheese, Chevre

- Chewing gum

- Chickpeas

- Chickory root

- Chocolate

- Powdered cocoa

- Instant coffee

- Coffee substitutes

- Cooking oils

- Cordials

- Fresh/frozen/canned corn

- Cornstarch

- Corn syrup

- Cheese, cottage

- Cottonseed

- Couscous

- Lactose-containing cream

- Cream of tartar

- Cheese, cream

- Commercial dextrose

- Soft drinks

- Beans, faba

- Cheese, feta

- Smoked fish

- Preserved fish

- Salted fish

- Breaded fish

- Canned fish with sauces

- Grain flour

- Fructo-oligosaccharides

- Fructose

- Canned fruit

- Preserved fruit

- Beans, garbanzo

- Cheese, Gjetost

- All kinds of grains

- Cheese, Gruyere

- Ham

- Hotdogs

- Commercial ice cream

- Jams

- Jellies

- Artichoke, Jerusalem

- Commercial ketchup

- Lactose

- Liquors

- Margarines

- Butter replacements

- Processed meats

- Preserved meats

- Smoked meats

- Salted meats

- Millet

- Canned coconut milk

- Soy milk

- Rice milk

- Cow's milk

- Dried milk

- Molasses

- Cheese, Mozzarella

- Beans, mung

- Cheese, Neufchatel

- Aspartame

- Salted nuts

- Roasted nuts

- Coated nuts

- Oats

- Okra

* Parsnips

* All kinds of pasta

* Pectin

* Postum

* White potatoes

* Sweet potatoes

* Cheese, Primost

* Quinoa

* Rice

* Cheese, ricotta

* Rye

* Saccharin

* Sago

* Commercial sausages

* Semolina

* Sherry

- Soda

- Commercial sour cream

- Soy

- Spelt

- All types of starch

- All kinds of sugar

- Tapioca

- Instant tea

- Instant coffee

- Triticale

- Turkey loaf

- Canned vegetables

- Preserved vegetables

- Wheat

- Wheat germ

- Powdered whey

- Liquid whey

- Yams

- Commercial yogurt

Next we will go through the GAPS Diet Approved Recipes.

12 - Breakfast

Nutty Coconut Granola

Ingredients:

- Pumpkin seeds, sprouted, chopped coarsely (1/4 cup)

- Almonds, chopped coarsely (1 cup)

- Pecans, chopped coarsely (1/4 cup)

- Cashews, chopped coarsely (1/4 cup)

- Walnuts, chopped coarsely (1/4 cup)

- Cinnamon, ground (1 teaspoon)

- Brown rice syrup (3 tablespoons)

- Coconut flakes, unsweetened (3 cups)

- Chia seeds (2 tablespoons)

- Coconut oil, melted (5 tablespoons)

Directions:

1. Set the oven at 250 degrees.

2. Meanwhile, use baking paper to line a large baking

sheet.

3. Place the pumpkin seeds, chia seeds, nuts, and the rest of the ingredients in a large bowl. Toss well until combined.

4. Pour the nut mixture onto the line sheet, making sure to spread evenly with a spatula.

5. Place in the oven to bake for about fifteen to twenty minutes or until golden brown on top.

6. Take out of the oven and let cool for ten minutes before serving.

Cheddar Nettle Omelet

Ingredients:

- Sea salt, unrefined (1/2 teaspoon)

- Heavy cream (1/4 cup)

- Chives, fresh, snipped finely (2 tablespoons)

- Stinging nettle leaves (8 ounces)

- Eggs (6 pieces)

- Butter/ghee, clarified (2 tablespoons)

- Cheddar cheese, sharp, thinly sliced (2 ounces)

Directions:

1. Fill a stockpot (medium) with the nettle leaves. Add water (1-2 tablespoons) and salt. Cover and heat on medium-low.

2. Remove from heat after twenty minutes or once the nettles are wilted. Transfer the nettle leaves into a sieve (fine mesh). Use the back of a large spoon to firmly press them. Once all their juices are released, set aside in a small bowl.

3. Place the eggs in a large bowl. Add heavy cream and beat until loosely mixed but not frothy. Set aside.

4. Meanwhile, heat a large skillet (cast iron) on medium-high before adding the butter. Once the butter is melted, add the egg mixture. Spread evenly on the pan and cook for five to ten seconds or until the edges start curling. Turn heat down to low before covering the pan and allowing the eggs to cook for an additional twenty to thirty seconds or until set.

5. Add the wilted nettles, chives, and cheddar cheese slices on top of one side of the cooked omelet. Fold and cover the pan again; allow to cook for twenty to thirty seconds more.

6. Serve immediately.

Cinnapple Pancakes

Ingredients:

- Applesauce (2 tablespoons)

- Baking soda (1/2 teaspoon)

- Coconut flour (1/2 cups)

- Cinnamon (1 tablespoon)

- Eggs, large (4 pieces)

- Honey (1 tablespoon)

- Sea salt, unrefined (1/2 teaspoon)

- Coconut oil – to be used in cooking the pancakes

Directions:

- Place the eggs in the food processor. Add the honey and applesauce, then process until just about combined.

- Gradually add the baking soda, salt, and coconut flour as you process the mixture again. Make sure the batter turns out colloidal in consistency (firm but still liquid).

- Meanwhile, heat a large pan on medium-low. Add the coconut oil/ghee; once heated, pour in the batter (1 heaping tablespoon) and cook for two to three minutes or until the bottom is browned. Sprinkle the pancake with cinnamon before flipping to cook on the other side for about two minutes. Repeat with the remaining batter.

- Place on a large plate. Top with yogurt and fruit.

- Serve and enjoy.

Breakfast Cookies

Ingredients:

- Cinnamon (1 ½ teaspoons)

- Almond butter (1/2 cup)

- Sea salt, unrefined (1/4 teaspoon)

- Cherries, dried (2 tablespoons)

- Applesauce, unsweetened (1/2 cup)

- Walnuts, chopped (2 tablespoons)

- Coconut flour (1/4 cup)

- Dates, pitted, pre-soaked for 15 min. in warm water (6 pieces)

- Eggs, beaten (2 pieces)

- Vanilla extract, pure (1 teaspoon)

- Baking soda (1/2 teaspoon)

- Currants (3 tablespoons)

Directions:

1. Set the oven at 350 degrees to preheat. Meanwhile, use parchment paper to line a large baking tray.

2. Fill the food processor with the dates, almond butter, and coconut flour. Process until the mixture is well-

blended, with the dates being ground to bits.

3. Pour in the eggs as well as the applesauce, shredded coconut, vanilla, baking soda, cinnamon, and salt. Process for half a minute or until you have a wet dough.

4. Toss in the rest of the ingredients and pulse a few times or until evenly combined.

5. Take a heaping spoonful of the dough and form into a ball before placing on the lined baking tray. Press lightly on the dough ball to form a circle. Do the same with the remaining batter.

6. Place in the oven to bake for about twelve to fifteen minutes or until the top of each cookie is golden and their edges are a bit browned.

7. Let cool for about fifteen to twenty minutes, then serve.

Crumbly Almond Blueberry Breakfast Muffins

Ingredients:

- Blueberries (1 cup)

- Coconut flour (1/2 cup)

- Sea salt, unrefined (1/2 teaspoon)

- Honey (1/2 cup)

- Butter (1 tablespoon)

- Almond flour, divided (2 cups)

- Eggs, pasture-raised (6 pieces)

- Vanilla, pure (3/4 teaspoon)

- Butter/coconut oil – to be used in greasing the muffin pan

Directions:

1. Set the oven at 350 degrees to preheat.

2. Meanwhile, use butter/coconut oil to generously coat 8 muffin cups. Set aside.

3. Reserve 2 tablespoons worth of almond flour. Place the rest in a large bowl and combine with salt and coconut flour. Set aside.

4. Place the eggs in another large bowl. Add the vanilla and honey, then whisk until combined. Pour the egg mixture into the flour mixture and stir to combine.

5. Add the blueberries to the batter and gently fold in. Pour into the greased muffin cups, patting down on top to form rounded heaps. Brush a bit of butter on top of each cup, then sprinkle with the reserved almond flour.

6. Place in the oven and bake for about thirty to forty minutes or until firm yet springy on top.

7. Serve and enjoy.

Cream Cheese & Carrot Morning Cupcakes

Ingredients:

- Baking soda (1 teaspoon)

- Coconut oil (1 cup)

- Coconut flour (1/2 cup)

- Carrots, scraped, grated (1 pound)

- Vanilla extract (2 teaspoons)

- Yogurt, full fat, warmed to room temp. (1/2 cup)

- Eggs, large, warmed to room temp. (4 pieces)

- Heavy cream, whipped (1 cup)

- Almond flour, blanched (2 cups)

- Sea salt, unrefined (1/2 teaspoon)

- Honey, divided (1 cup)

- Cream cheese (3/4 pound)

Directions:

1. Set the oven at 375 degrees to preheat after placing the rack in the middle.

2. Meanwhile, use muffin liners to line 24 muffin cups. Set aside.

3. Place the almond flour, coconut flour, salt, baking soda, and baking powder in a large bowl. Beat on low for twenty seconds before adding in the grated carrots. Beat for another half a minute or until mixture is evenly combined.

4. Fill a blender with the eggs as well as honey (3/4 cup). Process for about twenty seconds and then pour in the yogurt and coconut oil. Process for twenty seconds more or until the mixture is well-blended and smooth.

5. Add the egg mixture to the flour mixture and lightly beat until mixed. Transfer the batter onto the lined muffin cups, making sure each cup is ¾ full.

6. Place in the oven to bake for about eighteen to twenty minutes or until golden brown on the edges. Allow the cupcakes to completely cool down.

7. Place the cream cheese as well as the remaining honey (1/4 cup) and vanilla in a large bowl. Whisk until the mixture is smooth, and then gently fold in the whipped cream.

8. Cover the top of each cooled cupcake with the pre-pared frosting.

9. Serve and enjoy.

13 - Lunch

Tarragon & Mustard Chicken

Ingredients:

- White wine, dry (1/2 cup)

- Mustard, Dijon-style (2 tablespoons)

- Heavy cream (1/2 cup)

- Chicken broth, homemade (2 cups)

- Butter, melted (2 tablespoons)

- Sea salt (1/4 teaspoon)

- Black pepper, freshly ground (1/4 teaspoon)

- Chicken, whole, pasture-raised (1 piece)

- Tarragon, fresh (5 sprigs)

Directions:

1. Set the oven at 400 degrees to preheat.

2. Remove the breastbone from the chicken. Slice the chicken breasts into halves and place on a roasting pan (stainless steel) with their skin side up. (Set aside

the neck and back in a large bowl for using later in making the stock.)

3. Pour the melted butter into a small bowl. Add the mustard and mix well with the butter. Brush this mixture on the chicken skin before sprinkling with pepper and salt.

4. Top the chicken pieces with tarragon, then place in the oven to bake for one hour or until the meat is completely cooked and the skin is golden brown. Transfer the cooked chicken pieces onto a platter; cover with foil to keep warm and set aside.

5. Heat the baking pan on medium. Add the wine for deglazing. Stir in the broth, then allow the mixture to boil. Once the mixture is reduced by ½ its original volume, gradually stir in the cream. Allow the entire mixture to boil for a few minutes more or until thickened to your desired consistency.

6. Season the prepared sauce with salt, then strain into a gravy boat. Serve alongside the chicken and enjoy.

Savory Onion Soup

Ingredients:

- Red onions, peeled, sliced thinly (3/4 pound)

- Beef stock (1 ½ quarts)

- Bay leaves (2 pieces)

- Gruyere cheese, shredded (4 ounces)

- Shallots, peeled, sliced thinly (1/4 pound)

- White wine, dry (1 cup)

- Thyme (3 sprigs)

- Black peppercorns, smoked (1 teaspoon)

- Sourdough bread, day old (4 slices)

- Beef tallow, grass-fed (1 tablespoon)

- Yellow onions, peeled, thinly sliced (1 pound)

- Sea salt, unrefined (1 teaspoon)

Directions:

1. Heat a stock pot (heavy-bottomed) on medium-high. Add the tallow and allow to melt before stirring in the shallots and onions.

2. Turn heat down to medium-low. Add the salt and stir to combine. Cover the pot and allow the shallots and onions to sweat for about ten minutes or until translucent and softened.

3. Place the peppercorns, thyme, and bay leaves inside a muslin bag or cheesecloth. Secure with kitchen twine and add to the bottom of the pot. Pour in the wine and beef stock.

4. Allow the mixture to simmer (without covering the pot) for about twenty to thirty minutes or until the liquid is already 1/3 its original volume.

5. Meanwhile, set the oven at 350 degrees to preheat.

6. Once the soup is done, transfer into soup bowls (ovenproof). Add a piece of sourdough bread (day-old) on top, then sprinkle with shredded cheese (1 ounce).

7. Cover and place in the oven to bake for twenty

minutes or until heated through and the cheese is melted.

8. Serve immediately.

Mustard & Leek Carrot Soup

Ingredients:

- Chicken broth, fresh (1 ½ quarts)

- Butter (1 tablespoon)

- Milk, whole (1 cup)

- Carrots, medium, scraped, chopped into quarter-inch thick circles (12 pieces)

- Chives, chopped (1 tablespoon)

- Mustard seeds (2 tablespoons)

- Leek, large, white/green, thinly sliced (1 piece)

- Sea salt, unrefined (1 teaspoon)

- Sour cream (1 dollop)

Directions:

1. Heat a stock pot (heavy-bottomed) on high before adding in the mustard seeds. Cover and cook until popping, then turn heat down to medium-low.

2. Add the butter and stir to combine with the popped mustard seeds. Once the butter is melted, add the carrots and leeks. Sprinkle with salt and stir before covering again. Allow the vegetables to sweat for four minutes or until the leeks have softened.

3. Turn heat up to medium-high before adding the chicken broth. Cover and allow the entire mixture to simmer for about thirty minutes, then remove from heat.

4. Use an immersion blender to process the mixture until well-blended and smooth. Add the milk and a bit of salt, then give the mixture a good stir.

5. Pour the soup into individual bowls. Top with homemade yogurt or sour cream (a dollop) as well as fresh chives.

6. Serve and enjoy.

Steak with Wild Mushroom Sauce

Ingredients:

Steak:

- Sea salt, unrefined (1/2 teaspoon)

- Beef, grass fed (1 pound)

- Black pepper, freshly ground (1/2 teaspoon)

- Shallots, minced finely (2 pieces)

- Butter/ghee, clarified (2 tablespoons)

- Egg yolk, beaten (1 piece)

Sauce:

- Butter/ghee, clarified, divided (1/4 cup)

- Beef stock, homemade (2 cups)

- Mushrooms, wild, coarsely chopped (3/4 pound)

- Red wine, dry (2 cups)

- Yellow onion, large, peeled, sliced thinly (1 piece)

- Thyme, fresh (2 sprigs)

Directions:

1. Place the ground beef in a large bowl. Add the minced shallots and combine roughly with the meat.

2. Add pepper, salt, and beaten egg to the beef mixture. Gently fold in to get everything well-mixed, then mold into 4 patties. Place on a large plate and set aside.

3. Pour the beef stock into a large pot. Add the fresh thyme and red wine; stir to combine. Heat on medium-high and allow to simmer until reduced to ½ of the original volume. Discard the thyme before adding butter (2 tablespoons); stir and allow mixture to simmer for about two minutes.

4. Meanwhile, heat a skillet (cast iron) on medium. Add the clarified butter (2 tablespoons) and allow to melt. Once butter is frothy, add the onions and sauté until fragrant and caramelized. Transfer the onions into a small bowl.

5. Add the mushrooms to the same skillet. Sauté until

fragrant and browned and then set aside in another bowl.

6. Add more clarified butter (2 tablespoons) to the skillet. Once melted, add the prepared patties and cook until just about done on both sides. Top with the onions and mushrooms before pouring on the prepared reduction sauce.

7. Simmer for several minutes more or until the meat is completely cooked. Transfer onto a platter and serve immediately.

Beef & Root Veggies Stew

Ingredients:

- Russet potatoes, medium, peeled, cubed (4 pieces)

- Sea salt, unrefined (1 teaspoon)

- Thyme leaves, fresh (1 tablespoon)

- Butter (1 tablespoon)

- Black pepper, freshly ground (1/2 teaspoon)

- Pearl onions (1 cup)

- Beef chuck roast, w/ sinew & excess fat trimmed (1 ½ pounds)

- Beef stock, homemade (1 quart)

- Bacon, chopped (8 ounces)

- Carrots, medium, scraped, chopped into quarter-inch thick circles (4 pieces)

- Red wine (1 ½ cups)

Directions:

1. Place the beef in a large bowl, season with pepper and salt, and set aside.

2. Heat a stock pot (heavy-bottomed) on medium-high before adding the butter. Once melted, stir in the bacon and cook until lightly browned and its fat is rendered.

3. Add the seasoned ground beef and stir with the bacon. Cook for tree minutes on each side.

4. Pour in the wine and stock. Add the vegetables as well and stir to combine.

5. Allow the mixture to boil before reducing heat to low. Cover and simmer for about four to five hours or until the beef is tenderized.

6. Transfer the cooked beef onto a large plate. Use two forks to shred the meat, then add back to the pot. Turn heat back up to medium-high, then allow everything to simmer until reduced to about a third of its original volume.

7. Serve topped with fresh thyme and enjoy.

Dill-Onion Chicken Roast

Ingredients:

- Onion, flowering (1 bunch)

- Sea salt, unrefined (1 teaspoon)

- Green garlic, chopped (4 heads)

- Dill, flowering (1 bunch)

- Red onions, young, chopped (1 bunch)

- Chicken, whole, w/ offal & giblets discarded (1 piece)

- Black pepper, freshly ground (1/2 teaspoon)

- Butter/ghee, clarified (1/4 cup)

- Lemons, large, quartered (2 pieces)

Directions:

1. Use wood/coal to set up a campfire, letting it burn white hot.

2. Meanwhile, use foil to line a single layer of parchment paper. Place the chicken on top and sprinkle with black pepper and salt. Set aside.

3. Mince ½ each of the flowering dill and onion. Add the chopped garlic and ghee or butter. Combine everything and spread on the chicken breast and skin. Drizzle the entire chicken with the juice from the lemon before stuffing its cavity with the rest of the onions, dill, and garlic as well as the used up lemons.

4. Use parchment paper to securely cover the entire chicken before covering again with foil (3 to 4 layers should do), making sure that no part of the chicken's skin comes in contact with the foil.

5. Cook the chicken in the campfire for about two hours or until evenly cooked on all sides. Once cooked, let it sit for fifteen to twenty minutes.

6. Discard the wrappings and serve the roasted chicken.

Lemon Sole

Ingredients:

- Flour, nut/sprouted (1/2 cup)

- Lemon juice, freshly squeezed (3 tablespoons)

- Lemon zest, freshly grated (3 tablespoons)

- Lemon slices (3 pieces)

- Butter/ghee, grass fed, divided (6 tablespoons)

- Parsley, fresh, curly, minced (3/4 cup)

- Sea salt, unrefined (1/4 teaspoon)

- Black pepper, freshly ground (1/4 teaspoon)

- Sole filets, Dover, 4-oz. (4 pieces)

Directions:

1. Place flour in a medium bowl. Add the filets and dredge until evenly coated on all sides. Transfer the coated filets on a large plate and set aside.

2. Meanwhile, heat a skillet (cast iron) on medium before adding the butter/ghee. Once the fat is melted, turn heat down to medium-low. Add the floured filets and cook for two minutes on each side. Transfer the cooked chicken onto a platter; set aside.

3. Add butter/ghee to the same skillet and allow to melt. Stir in the minced parsley, lemon juice, and lemon zest. Cook for an additional minute before pouring over the sole filets.

4. Sprinkle pepper and salt over the fish, top with lemon wedges, and serve immediately.

14 - Dinner

Coconut Lemongrass Chicken Soup

Ingredients:

- Lime leaves (6 pieces)

- Chicken stock, homemade (4 cups)

- Cilantro, fresh (5 sprigs)

- Thai basil, fresh (a handful)

- Ginger, 1", sliced, w/ peel reserved (2 pieces)

- Palm sugar (1 tablespoon)

- Lime wedges (2 pieces)

- Lemongrass stalk, 6", smashed (1 piece)

- Shiitake mushrooms, sliced thinly, w/ stems reserved (1/2 pound)

- Thai chilies, smashed (3 pieces)

- Coconut milk, full fat (13 ½ ounces)

- Shallots, peeled, diced, w/ skins reserved (2 pieces)

- Chicken thighs, skinless, boneless (1 ½ pounds)

- Fish sauce, reduced sodium (1/4 cup)

Directions:

1. Fill a large saucepan with the stock. Heat on medium and allow to simmer.

2. Add the shallot skins, lemongrass, shiitake stems, lime leaves, ginger peelings, and chilies. Stir to combine before covering the pan. Allow the mixture to cook for twenty minutes or until all flavors are well-blended.

3. Remove broth from the heat once done. Strain into a large jar, making sure no stray solids are included.

4. Meanwhile, wipe clean the pan. Pour in the strained broth, fish sauce, and coconut milk, as well as the palm sugar, shallots, ginger, and mushroom caps. Stir to combine and then add the chicken thighs.

5. Allow the entire mixture to simmer on medium for twenty-five to thirty minutes or until the chicken is opaque white and completely cooked.

6. Divide the soup among individual bowls and top with Thai basil, cilantro sprigs, and lime wedges.

7. Serve and enjoy.

Veggie Seafood Stew

Ingredients:

Broth:

- Seafood broth, warm (6 cups)

- Chiles, red/green, fresh (2 pieces)

- Sea salt, unrefined (1/4 teaspoon)

- Garlic, chopped finely (2 tablespoons)

- White onion, small, thinly sliced (1 piece)

- Red pepper paste, Korean (1 tablespoon)

- Ginger, chopped finely (3/4 tablespoon)

- Honey (1 teaspoon)

- Lard (4 tablespoons)

- Scallions, white portion, thinly sliced (5 pieces)

- Red pepper flakes, Korean (1 tablespoon)

- Fish sauce (3 tablespoons)

Veggies:

- Shiitake mushrooms, medium, chopped into quarter-inch thick slices (3 pieces)

- Pea shoots (a handful)

- Enoki mushrooms, trimmed of roots, separated (a handful)

- Scallion greens, chopped into two-inch portions (a handful)

- White radishes, young, small, chopped into quarter-inch thick slices (2 pieces)

- Carrot, medium, chopped into quarter-inch thick slices (1 piece)

- Baby tatsoi (4 pieces)

- Watercress (1/2 bunch)

Seafood:

- Shrimp (1 pound)

- White fish, firm, cubed (1 pound)

- Clams (1 pound)

Garnish:

- Mung bean sprouts, fresh (a handful)

- Cilantro, fresh, chopped roughly (a handful)

- Chile, sliced (1 tablespoon)

Directions:

1. Heat a large, heavy bottomed pot on medium-high. Add the lard and allow it to melt before stirring in the onion, scallion, and chili. Fry for about three to four minutes or until lightly browned.

2. Stir in the ginger as well as garlic; cook for two minutes or until fragrant. Pour in the warm broth and give everything a good stir. Allow the mixture to simmer before adding in the honey, Korean pepper flakes & paste, and fish sauce. Stir to combine and allow to boil.

3. Once boiling, stir in the carrots, baby tatsoi, radish, enoki, and shiitake. Boil for one minute more before reducing heat to low. Cover and cook for another fifteen minutes or until the vegetables are softened.

4. Stir in the reserved green scallions, watercress, and pea shoots. Allow the entire mixture to simmer on medium for about five minutes, then reduce heat back to low.

5. Stir in the clams and shrimps. Cover and cook until clams are opened, then stir in the fish chunks. Simmer for about four to five minutes more, then transfer into bowls.

6. Serve immediately with rice.

Easy Burger Salads

Ingredients:

- Pickles, sour, medium, chopped into quarter-inch circles (2 pieces)

- Beef, grass-fed, ground (1 pound)

- Salad greens, packed loosely (6 cups)

- Cheese, grass-fed, shredded (4 ounces)

- Tomatoes, chopped (1/2 pound)

- Bacon fat (1 tablespoon)

- White onion, small, thinly sliced (1 piece)

- Mayonnaise, homemade (1 tablespoon)

- Ketchup, homemade (1 tablespoon)

Directions:

1. Heat a skillet (heavy-bottomed) on medium-high. Add the lard/bacon fat, then the ground beef. Cook until the meat is browned.

2. Transfer the cooked ground beef into a serving bowl. Let sit to cool for five minutes.

3. Arrange the greens on a large plate. Add the ground beef on top.

4. Garnish with onion, tomatoes, pickles, and cheese.

5. Top with a dollop each of ketchup and mayonnaise.

6. Serve right away.

Red Wine Bison Stew

Ingredients:

- Sea salt, unrefined (1/2 teaspoon)

- Yellow onion, small, chopped finely (1 piece)

- Potatoes, medium, peeled, chopped into 1" cubes (3 pieces)

- Bay leaves (2 pieces)

- Bacon fat (2 tablespoons)

- Red wine (2 cups)

- Thyme (2 sprigs)

- Tomato paste (1/2 cup)

- Black pepper, freshly ground (1/2 teaspoon)

- Carrots, chopped into quarter-inch thick circles (3 pieces)

- Beef stock, homemade (2 cups)

- Parsley, chopped (3 tablespoons)

- Bison stew meat (1 pound)

- Rosemary (1 branch)

- Celery ribs, finely chopped (3 pieces)

Directions:

1. Place the meat in a large bowl. Sprinkle pepper and salt on the meat and let sit.

2. Heat a cast iron skillet oven on medium-high before adding the bacon fat. Stir in the thyme and rosemary; cook for about two to three minutes, then discard.

3. Add the seasoned bison stew meat and cook for about five minutes on both sides or until nicely seared. Once done, transfer onto a plate and set aside.

4. Add the carrots, onion, and celery to the same pan. Cook for about five to six minutes or until tenderly crisp. Add the meat back in the pan; add the potatoes as well.

5. Add the red wine, beef stock, and tomato paste; stir everything to combine. Add the bay leaves before covering the pan and allowing the entire mixture to sim-

mer for about two hours on medium-low.

6. Discard the bay leaves before placing the stew in individual bowls. Top with chopped parsley and serve immediately.

Walnut Beet Salad

Ingredients:

Salad:

- Red onion, small, chopped into 1/8-inch rings (1 piece)

- Butter, clarified (1 tablespoon)

- Beets (2 pounds)

- Walnuts, chopped (3/4 cup)

Dressing:

- Sea salt, unrefined, finely ground (1/4 teaspoon)

- Allspice, ground (1/4 teaspoon)

- Walnut oil, cold pressed (2 tablespoons)

- Kombucha (2 tablespoons)

- Cloves, ground (1/8 teaspoon)

- Olive oil, extra virgin (2 tablespoons)

Directions:

1. Set the oven at 425 degrees to preheat.

2. Meanwhile, remove the tops and root tips off the beets. Brush each beet with a little clarified butter before wrapping in parchment paper and aluminum foil.

3. Place in the oven to roast for about forty-five minutes to one hour or until tender. Once the beets are done, place in the refrigerator for eight to twenty-four hours.

4. Pour the kombucha tea in a medium bowl. Add the olive oils, salt, cloves, walnut, and allspice. Stir to combine, then set aside in the refrigerator.

5. Heat a skillet on medium-high. Once hot, add the walnuts and toss for about three to five minutes or until nicely toasted. Transfer into a large bowl and set

aside to cool.

6. Chop the chilled beets into cubes and add to the toasted walnuts. Add the sliced onion as well, then toss everything to combine.

7. Drizzle salad with the prepared dressing. Toss gently and serve immediately.

Smokin' Salmon Roe

Ingredients:

- Salmon roe, wild caught, w/ skeins intact (3 pounds)

- Sea salt, unrefined (1/4 cup)

Directions:

1. Rinse the roe skeins with filtered water. Meanwhile, preheat the smoker.

2. Pat dry and lightly coat with sea salt. Place in a large bowl to cure for about thirty minutes.

3. Drain extra moisture and brush off extra salt from the roe skeins, then place in the preheated smoker. Cook for about thirty to forty-five minutes.

4. Once cooked, place in the refrigerator to chill.

5. Serve with greens or eggs. Enjoy.

Tasty Rosemary Steak

Ingredients:

- Rosemary, fresh (1 branch)

- Rosemary, fresh, chopped finely (1 tablespoon)

- Butter, clarified (2 tablespoons)

- Sea salt, unrefined (1/4 teaspoon)

- Black pepper, freshly ground (1/4 teaspoon)

- Garlic cloves, chopped finely (6 pieces)

- Red wine (1 cup)

- Beef steak, grass fed (16 ounces)

Directions:

1. Set the oven at 300 degrees to preheat.

2. Season the steak generously with sea salt and black pepper. Set aside.

3. Heat a skillet (cast iron) on medium-high before adding the butter. Once melted, add the steak and cook on each side for about one minute or until seared.

4. Transfer the seared steak on a platter; set aside. Meanwhile, stir the fresh rosemary needles and garlic to the same skillet. Add red wine to deglaze the pan, then return the steak and place in the oven for ten minutes.

5. Serve topped with more rosemary and enjoy.

15 - Condiments

Hot Garlic Kraut

Ingredients:

- Garlic cloves, minced (3 pieces)

- Sea salt, unrefined (1 tablespoon)

- Red cabbage, shredded (3 ½ pounds)

- Jalapeno pepper, medium, thinly sliced (4 pieces)

Directions:

1. Place the cabbage in a large bowl. Add the garlic, sea salt, and jalapenos, then toss to combine. Knead the mixture for about five minutes or until their juices are released. Let sit for another five minutes before kneading again for about five minutes.

2. Place the salted veggies at the bottom of a fermentation jar, making sure they are arranged in layers. Make sure they are packed firmly and completely submerged in liquid.

3. Cover and leave the jar at room temperature to allow the vegetables to ferment for about three to four

weeks.

4. Place in the refrigerator, where it should keep for up to nine months.

Easy Green Chile Salsa

Ingredients:

- Jalapenos, deseeded, w/ stems removed (8 pieces)

- Cumin seeds, whole, roasted, crushed (2 tablespoons)

- Garlic cloves, large (8 pieces)

- Sea salt, finely ground (2 tablespoons)

- Green chili peppers, deseeded, w/ stems removed (8 pieces)

- Ancho peppers, deseeded, w/ stems removed (8 pieces)

- Onions, large (2 pieces)

- Coriander seeds, whole, roasted, crushed (2 tablespoons)

Directions:

1. Place the peppers, salt, and spices inside a food processor. Add the rest of the vegetables, then process until well blended.

2. Transfer the mashed mixture into 2 jars (quart-sized), making sure to about one inch of air space is left. Add weights before sealing the jars and leaving them at room temperature for ten days to three months. (The longer the veggies are left to ferment, the sourer and more flavorful they will turn out.)

3. Once the green peppers have achieved a muted olive green color, place in the refrigerator and use within a year.

GAPS-Friendly Pepperoncini

Ingredients:

- Sea salt, unrefined, finely ground (2 tablespoons)

- Pepperoncini peppers, fresh, whole, packed firmly (4 cups)

- Bay leaf (1 piece)

- Water, filtered (3 cups)

- Vegetable starter culture (1 package)

- Garlic cloves (2 pieces)

Directions:

1. Fill a saucepan (medium sized) with water and heat on medium-low. Once the temperature of the water reaches 100 degrees, add the salt and stir until completely dissolved.

2. Transfer the warm brine into a large pitcher. Let sit at room temperature to cool down before whisking in the vegetable starter culture.

3. Fill a fermentation jar (quart-size) with the pepperoncini, making sure they are packed but not bruised. Add the bay leaf as well as garlic cloves before pouring in the cooled brine.

4. Seal the jar and place in an area away from direct sunlight. Allow the pepperoncini to ferment at room temperature for about ten days or until their color turns into faded yellow.

5. Transfer the fermented pepperoncini in the refrigerator, where it should keep for up to one year.

No-Fuss Sauerkraut

Ingredients:

- Sea salt, unrefined (2 tablespoons)

- Cabbage heads, medium (2 pieces)

Directions:

1. Trim the cabbage of its core as well as any damaged leaves.

2. Chop the cabbage into long, 1/8-inch thick shredded pieces and place in a large bowl.

3. Add salt to the shredded cabbage. Toss to combine and let sit for five minutes or until the cabbage is softened and its juice is released.

4. Give the salted cabbage a good squeeze and then place in a vegetable fermenter. Pack tightly to remove air pockets and make sure the cabbage is fully submerged in liquid.

5. Seal the fermenter and let sit for one month to six months at room temperature.

6. Once fermented, transfer the sauerkraut into glass jars. Store in the refrigerator and use within one year.

Fennel & Cucumber Pickles

Ingredients:

- Pickling spice (2 tablespoons)

- Water (1/4 cup)

- Fennel bulb, medium, cored, sliced thinly (1 piece)

- Sea salt (3 tablespoons)

- Dill, flowering (1 head)

- Cane vinegar (3/4 cup)

- Honey (1/2 cup)

- Cucumbers, medium, peeled, sliced thinly (2 pieces)

- Bay leaf (2 pieces)

Directions:

1. Heat a saucepan filled with the water and vinegar on medium. Once the liquids are warmed, stir in the sea

salt, pickling spice, and honey.

2. Remove from heat once the mixture is fully blended.

3. Meanwhile, fill a glass jar (quart-sized) with the sliced fennel and cucumber. Add the dill and bay leaves on top before pouring in the seasoned vinegar.

4. Seal the jar and place in the refrigerator to chill for twenty-four hours.

5. Serve and enjoy.

16 - Spreads

Bacon-Shallot Potted Cheddar

Ingredients:

- Cheddar cheese, sharp, shredded (12 ounces)

- Ghee/butter, clarified, organic (2 tablespoons)

- Heavy cream (1 cup)

- Bacon (8 ounces)

- Sherry, dry (2 tablespoons)

- Shallots, medium, thinly sliced (2 pieces)

Directions:

1. Heat a pan on medium-high before adding the ghee.

2. Add the bacon and fry until completely cooked and nicely crisp.

3. Transfer the cooked bacon onto a large plate and allow to cool a bit. Discard the bacon fat in the pan, save for 2 tablespoons.

4. Turn the heat down to medium-low before adding the

shallots to the bacon fat. Sauté for about fifteen minutes or until browned and fragrant.

5. Meanwhile, place the cooled bacon in the food processor. Add the cheddar, then process until combined. Pour in the cream and sherry as well as the sautéed shallots. Process again until the mixture is smooth and spreadable in consistency.

6. Transfer the prepared cheese spread into ramekins or jars. Place in the refrigerator, where it will keep for up to one month.

7. To serve: Allow potted cheddar to warm to room temperature first. Spread on bread slices or crackers, and enjoy.

Homemade Avocado Oil Mayo

Ingredients:

- Water (1 tablespoon)

- Sea salt, coarsely ground (1/2 teaspoon)

- Egg yolks, duck (2 pieces) OR chicken (3 pieces)

- Lemon juice, freshly squeezed (2 tablespoons)

- Avocado oil (1 ½ cups)

Directions:

1. Place the egg yolks in a food processor. Sprinkle with salt, add in the lemon juice, and pour in the water.

2. Process until roughly combined, then gradually stream in the avocado oil as you process the mixture for two minutes or until thickened and well-blended.

3. Transfer the prepared mayonnaise into an airtight jar. Place in the refrigerator and use within one week.

Honey Whiskey Marmalade

Ingredients:

- Honey (1 quart)

- Seville oranges (8 pieces)

- Irish whiskey (1/2 cup)

Directions:

1. After scrubbing the oranges, place them inside the

pressure cooker.

2. Fill the bottom of the cooker with enough water to cover the oranges. Cook for about ten minutes or until softened, then turn the oranges. Cook for five more minutes or until the rinds of the oranges are evenly softened.

3. Remove the oranges and allow to cool on a plate. Once cooled, slice into crosswise halves. Remove the seeds before scooping out the pulp.

4. Place the orange pulp in the blender. Process until smooth, then transfer to a pot.

5. Slice the orange rinds into matchstick-sized pieces, then drop into the pot. Add the honey and stir with the orange pulp and rind until well-combined.

6. Heat the pot on medium-high and allow the mixture to boil before reducing heat to medium. Stir the mixture continuously for about thirty to thirty-five minutes or until set.

7. Remove the prepared marmalade from the heat and let cool for about five minutes. Stir the whiskey into

the marmalade before placing in airtight glass jars.

8. Process the marmalade in the water bath. After ten minutes, remove and serve or store in the refriger-ator.

Easy Sage Pate

Ingredients:

- Milk, fresh (1 quart)

- Shallots, large, chopped finely (2 pieces)

- Sherry (1/2 cup)

- Chicken livers (1 pound)

- Ghee, grass fed (14 ounces) OR butter (8 ounces) + ghee (6 ounces)

- Sage, rubbed (2 tablespoons)

- Sage leaves, fresh (1 tablespoon)

Directions:

1. Rinse, drain, and place the chicken livers in a large bowl.

2. Add the fresh milk, making sure the chicken livers are fully covered. Let sit to marinate for four to twenty-four hours.

3. Rinse the marinated chicken livers after draining, then set aside in a medium bowl.

4. Meanwhile, heat a large skillet on medium-high before adding the ghee (4 ounces). Once the ghee has melted, stir in the sliced shallots. Cook until browned, then stir in the chicken livers.

5. Allow the chicken livers to simmer in their own juices, then cook further for several minutes or until the liquid is evaporated and the chicken livers are crumbling into bits.

6. Stir in the rubbed sage, then pour in the sherry to deglaze the skillet. Cook for a few minutes or until the sherry has evaporated. Let sit to cool.

7. Transfer the cooked chicken liver mixture into the food processor. Add softened ghee or butter (8 ounces) and process until well-blended and smooth.

8. Heat another skillet on medium before adding the re-

maining ghee (2 ounces). Turn off the heat once the ghee has melted.

9. Divide the prepared pâté among individual bowls. Top with fresh sage before pouring on the melted ghee.

10. Place in the refrigerator to chill overnight; warm to room temperature before serving.

11. Enjoy.

Delish Dill Mayo

Ingredients:

- Vinegar, white wine (2 tablespoons)

- Cayenne pepper (a dash)

- Olive oil, extra virgin, unrefined (1/2 cup)

- Egg yolk (1 piece)

- Dill, fresh, snipped (1/4 cup)

- Sea salt, unrefined (a dash)

Directions:

1. Place the egg yolk in the food processor.

2. Add the fresh dill, unrefined sea salt, cayenne pepper, and vinegar.

3. Pulse several times until all ingredients are blended.

4. Gradually stream in the olive oil as you process the mixture for one minute or until creamy and well-emulsified.

5. Place in the refrigerator.

17 - Beverages

Kombucha Cranberry Slushy

Ingredients:

- Kombucha tea (1 ½ cups)

- Honey (1 tablespoon)

- Cranberry juice (2 cups)

- Lime (1 piece)

- Cranberries, fresh (1 cup)

Directions:

1. Place the cranberries in the blender.

2. Pour in the kombucha tea as well as the honey and juice from the lime.

3. Process for half a minute or until well-blended and the cranberries are broken into bits.

4. Serve and enjoy.

Nourishing Ginger Tea

Ingredients:

- Ginger, fresh, ½" (1 knob)

- Coconut milk, full fat (1 cup)

- Manuka honey (1 tablespoon)

- Turmeric, fresh, 1" (1 knob)

- Ghee (1 teaspoon)

- Coconut water (1 cup)

Directions:

1. After peeling off the skins, grate the ginger and turmeric into fine bits.

2. Add the ghee and grind until the mixture turns into a fine paste.

3. Transfer the paste into a large saucepan. Pour in the coconut water and coconut milk. Heat on medium-high and cook until the mixture starts bubbling at the sides.

4. Cover the pan and remove from the heat. Let the mixture steep for three minutes before straining.

5. Transfer to a teapot and add the honey. Stir to com-

bine and serve right away.

Gut-Friendly Soda

Ingredients:

- Honey (1 cup)

- Whey, fresh (1/2 cup)

- Water (6 cups)

- Lemon juice, freshly squeezed (1 cup)

Directions:

1. Heat a saucepan filled with water on low. Add the honey and whisk until completely dissolved.

2. Remove from the heat and add the whey as well as lemon juice. Whisk again to combine before pouring into clean bottles (flip-top).

3. After sealing the bottles, place on the counter to ferment at room temperature for four to seven days or until sour and fizzy.

4. Serve and enjoy.

Fermented Green Tea

Ingredients:

- Green tea, loose leaf (2 teaspoons)

- Jun culture (1 piece)

- Water, filtered (8 cups)

- Honey, raw (1/2 cup)

- Jun tea (1/2 cup)

Directions:

1. Fill a kettle with water and heat to 165 degrees.

2. Meanwhile, place the green tea leaves at the bottom of a large pitcher. Add the hot water. Allow the tea leaves to steep for two minutes before straining into a mason jar.

3. Stir in the honey, then allow the tea mixture to cool before dumping in the Jun culture. Leave the jar for three days at room temperature.

4. Strain the tea mixture into 4 bottles (flip-top). Seal

and allow to ferment again for about two to three days.

5. Drink away, or chill before serving.

Lime Apple Tonic

Ingredients:

- Limes, medium (2 pieces)

- Parsley, fresh (1 ounce)

- Marine collagen (2 tablespoons)

- Apples, medium, Granny Smith (3 pieces)

- Mint, fresh (1 ounce)

- Wheatgrass (1/2 ounce)

Directions:

1. Chop the apples roughly and place in the blender.

2. Place the lime (discard the rind) in the blender as well after chopping to bits.

3. Add the wheatgrass, parsley, and mint to the apples

and lime. Process until well-blended.

4. Pour the mixture into a large pitcher. Add the collagen peptides and stir to combine.

5. Serve immediately.

Heartwarming Mulled Wine

Ingredients:

- Red wine (1 bottle)

- Nutmeg pod, small (1 piece)

- Apple cider, sweet (6 cups)

- Black peppercorns (8 pieces)

- Anise seeds (1 teaspoon)

- Honey (1 cup)

- Cinnamon sticks (2 pieces)

- Bay leaves (2 pieces)

- Cloves, whole (6 pieces)

- Cardamom pods (8 pieces)

- Fennel seeds (1 teaspoon)

- Brandy (1 cup)

- Oranges (2 pieces)

Directions:

1. Place the spices in the middle of a square cheesecloth. Secure with a kitchen twine and place inside a stock pot (nonreactive).

2. Add the honey, cider, brandy, and wine. Stir until combined, then add in 1 orange (sliced) as well as the bay leaves.

3. Heat the pot on low for one hour or until the flavors are well-blended. Add the remaining orange slices.

4. Serve warm and enjoy.

Invigorating Water Kefir

Ingredients:

For 1st fermentation:

- Cane sugar, organic (1/4 cup)

- Lemon, halved (1 piece)

- Water kefir grains (1/4 cup)

- Figs, unsulphured, dried (2 pieces)

For 2nd fermentation:

- Cane sugar, organic (2 tablespoons) OR fruit juice, 100% (1/2 cup)

Directions:

1. Fill a pot with filtered water (6 cups) and heat on medium-high. Allow the water to come to a boil before adding the sugar. Stir to dissolve the sugar completely. Turn off the heat and let the sugar mixture cool down.

2. Fill a glass jar (2-quart) with the grains (water kefir). Add the cooled sugar water as well as halved lemon and dried figs.

3. Securely cover the jar with a piece of cheesecloth and kitchen twine. Leave at room temperature to allow the water kefir to ferment for about two to three days.

4. Once the kefir is fermented enough to deliver the fla-

vor intensity you prefer, pass through a wooden strainer to remove the figs and lemon (set the grains aside in the refrigerator for re-culturing within a week).

5. Place the water kefir in the refrigerator to chill for two hours before serving. OR

6. You may ferment the water kefir a second time if you would prefer the drink to be fizzy. Simply fill a bottle (flip-top) with fruit juice (1/4 cup) or organic cane sugar (1 tablespoon), then pour in the water kefir (leave about one inch of head space).

7. Seal the bottle and leave to ferment at room temperature for eighteen to twenty-four hours. Place in the refrigerator to chill for three days or until the bubbles have settled. Serve and enjoy.

18 - Snacks And Treats

Blood Orange & Coconut Jelly-Mousse

Ingredients:

Jelly:

- Water, cold (1 tablespoon)

- Honey (1/3 cup)

- Blood orange juice (1 cup)

- Gelatin, unflavored (1 ½ teaspoons)

- Orange extract, organic (1/2 teaspoon)

Mousse:

- Gelatin, unflavored (1 tablespoon)

- Blood orange peel, grated finely (1 teaspoon)

- Honey (1/3 cup)

- Coconut milk, full fat (28 ounces)

- Vanilla extract, pure (1 teaspoon)

- Water, cold (3 tablespoons)

Toppings:

- Coconut flakes, unsweetened, dried (1/4 cup)

Directions:

1. Refrigerate the coconut milk for two to four hours or until the cream has separated from the milk (the hardened cream should have risen to the surface).

2. Reserve the cream in a covered bowl and place in the refrigerator. Meanwhile, transfer the coconut milk into a saucepan. Add the honey and whisk well until well-combined with the coconut milk. Heat the pan on medium and allow the coconut cream/honey mixture to come to a boil. Once the mixture is thickened and reduced to about ½ cup, remove from heat and let cool.

3. Meanwhile, fill a small bowl with gelatin (1 tablespoon) and cold water (3 tablespoons). Allow the gelatin to sit for one to two minutes or until softened and thickened with the consistency of applesauce.

4. Pour the softened gelatin into the pan containing the coconut milk/honey mixture. Whisk well to combine,

making sure there are no remaining lumps.

5. Place the refrigerated coconut cream in the mixing bowl. Add the vanilla and orange peel, then whisk at high speed until uniformly smooth and fluffed up.

6. Add the coconut milk to the whisked coconut cream and gently fold in. Do the same with the honey and remaining coconut milk.

7. Divide the prepared coconut mousse among individual dishes or glasses. Place in the refrigerator to chill for two hours or until set.

8. Meanwhile, fill a saucepan with blood orange juice and honey (1/3 cup). Stir to combine, then heat on medium-high. Allow the mixture to simmer for several minutes or until thickened and reduced to about ¾ its original volume. Remove from heat and set aside.

9. Place gelatin (1 ½ teaspoons) in a small bowl. Add cold water (1 tablespoon) and let sit until softened and as thick as applesauce. Pour this softened gelatin into the blood orange mixture; add the rosewater and orange extract as well.

10. Whisk well to combine, making sure the gelatin is completely dissolved and there are no lumps left. Stir and allow the entire mixture to sit for five minutes or until slightly cooled and can be easily poured.

11. Remove the coconut mousse-filled dishes or glasses from the refrigerator. Top each with the blood orange mixture, then place back in the refrigerator. Allow chilling for two hours or until set.

12. Heat a skillet (stainless steel) on medium, then add the coconut flakes. Stirring frequently, cook the coconut flakes until toasted and lightly browned.

13. Top each jelly-mousse with the toasted coconut flakes and serve immediately.

Nutty Strawberry Bowl with Yogurt

Ingredients:

- Fennel, ground (1/8 teaspoon)

- Honey (2 tablespoons)

- Pine nuts (1/4 cup)

- Coriander, ground (1/4 teaspoon)

- Yogurt, Greek style, strained (4 cups)

- Strawberries, fresh (12 ounces)

- Vanilla bean powder (1/4 teaspoon)

- Bee pollen (1 teaspoon)

- Mint leaves, fresh (6 pieces)

Directions:

1. Slice the strawberries into quarters after hulling them. Place in a large bowl.

2. Drizzle the strawberries with honey before sprinkling with fennel, coriander, and vanilla bean powder. Toss gently to combine, making sure the strawberries are evenly coated with honey.

3. Place the strawberry mixture in an airtight jar. Allow chilling overnight in the refrigerator.

4. Fill 4 individual bowls with yogurt. Add the strawberry mixture on top, then sprinkle with pine nuts and bee pollen. Garnish with mint (sliced thinly) and

serve.

5. Enjoy.

Creamy Coconut Ice Cream

Ingredients:

- Salt, unrefined (1/2 teaspoon)

- Cinnamon (1 teaspoon)

- Vanilla extract, pure (1 tablespoon)

- Nutmeg, ground (1/8 teaspoon)

- Cardamom, ground (1/8 teaspoon)

- Cloves, ground (1/8 teaspoon)

- Maple syrup, pure (1/2 cup)

- Coconut milk, full fat, canned (28 ounces)

Directions:

1. Place all ice cream ingredients in the blender. Process until the mixture is well-combined and smooth.

2. Follow the manufacturer's directions in processing

the ice cream mixture. OR

3. Place the blended ice cream mixture in an ice bath to chill. Meanwhile, place your ice cream container in the freezer for about two hours. Pour the ice cream mixture into the container and return to the freezer. Chill for forty-five minutes or until the mixture begins freezing near the edges.

4. Take out of the freezer and whisk vigorously with a spatula or handheld mixer, making sure any frozen sections are broken up. Place back in the freezer, then whisk again every thirty minutes thereafter. Repeat until your ice cream is all set and frozen.

Lemon-Thyme Toasted Almonds

Ingredients:

- Rosemary (1 branch)

- Almonds, blanched (2 cups)

- Sea salt, unrefined (1/2 teaspoon)

- Lard, pasture raised (1 tablespoon)

- Thyme, fresh (2 sprigs)

- Lemon zest, freshly grated (1/2 teaspoon)

Directions:

1. Heat a large skillet (cast iron) on medium-high before adding the lard.

2. Stir in the thyme and rosemary. Cook until the herbs are crisp and sizzling, then discard.

3. Add the almonds to the seasoned fat. Stir and cook until browned and fragrant.

4. Transfer the toasted almonds into a serving bowl. Add the lemon zest and salt, then gently toss to coat the almonds evenly.

5. Allow the toasted almonds to cool before serving.

Roasted Cabbage Wedges

Ingredients:

- Salt, kosher (1/4 teaspoon)

- Pepper, freshly cracked (1/4 teaspoon)

- Cabbage head, sliced into wedges (1 piece)

- Lemon juice, freshly squeezed (1 teaspoon)

- Olive oil, extra virgin (1 tablespoon)

Directions:

1. Set the oven at 375 degrees to preheat.

2. Chop the cabbage into wedged pieces, then arrange on a large baking sheet. Drizzle olive oil on the cabbage before seasoning with pepper and salt.

3. Place in the oven to roast for about twenty to thirty minutes or until golden brown and tender.

4. Serve sprinkled with lemon juice.

5. Enjoy.

Lentil Chili Snack

Ingredients:

- Yellow onion, medium, chopped finely (1 piece)

- Red pepper flakes, crushed (1 teaspoon)

- Sea salt, finely ground (1 tablespoon)

- Lentils, sprouted (16 ounces)

- Chile powder, mild (3 tablespoons)

- Bone broth, beef, long-simmered (8 cups)

- Olive oil, extra virgin (1/4 cup)

- Garlic cloves, chopped finely (6 pieces)

- Cumin, ground (1/4 cup)

- Oregano, dried (3 tablespoons)

- Cayenne pepper (1/4 teaspoon)

- Tomatoes, peeled, diced (3 cups)

Directions:

1. Heat a Dutch oven on medium-high. Add the olive oil, then stir in the garlic and onion. Sauté for three minutes or until translucent and fragrant.

2. Turn heat down to medium-low. Cook the garlic and onions for another ten minutes or until their edges are caramelized.

3. Add the spices and salt. Stir and cook for an additional one to two minutes.

4. Add the tomatoes and lentils. Stir as you add the broth. Allow the entire mixture to simmer on medium for fifteen minutes or until the lentils are fully cooked and tender.

5. Serve and enjoy.

Minty Strawberry Sorbet

Ingredients:

- Water (1/4 cup)

- Strawberries, hulled, fresh/frozen (6 cups)

- Vanilla extract, pure (1/2 teaspoon)

- Honey (3/4 cup)

- Mint, fresh (1 bunch)

- Lemon juice (1 tablespoon)

- Peppermint extract (1/4 teaspoon)

Directions:

1. Fill a saucepan with water and honey before heating on medium.

2. Add the mint, then remove the pan from the heat. Let the mint steep in the honey mixture as it cools down.

3. Strain the honey-mint mixture into a blender. Discard the mint before adding the strawberries, peppermint extract, vanilla, and lemon juice.

4. Process until mixture is well-blended and smooth, then strain into an airtight jar.

5. Place in the refrigerator to chill for eight hours or more or until completely cold.

6. Transfer into the ice cream maker; follow manufacturer's directions in processing the mixture into sorbet.

7. Serve and enjoy.

Honeyed Berry Mix

Ingredients:

- Honey (2 tablespoons)

- Sea salt (1/4 teaspoon)

- Berries, mixed (2 cups)

- Starter culture, packaged (1/2 teaspoon) OR whey, fresh (2 tablespoons)

Directions:

1. Fill a mason jar (pint size) with the berries. Use a wooden spoon to pack the berries firmly at the bottom; set aside.

2. Meanwhile, place the whey/starter culture in a large bowl. Add water (1 to 2 tablespoons), salt, and honey.

3. Pour the liquid into the jar, making sure the berries are completely submerged. Top up with water so that no air pockets remain.

4. Cover the jar and allow the berries to ferment at room temperature for one to two days.

5. Place in the refrigerator, where it will keep for one to two months.

19 - Baked Goods

Blueberry Banana Pudding

Ingredients:

- Coconut cream, organic (2 cups)

- Butter/ghee, organic (20 grams)

- Vanilla essence (1/2 teaspoon)

- Cinnamon (1 teaspoon)

- Yogurt, homemade (1 dollop)

- Banana bread (1/2 loaf)

- Blueberries (1 ½ cups)

- Eggs, free range, organic (2 pieces)

- Honey (1 tablespoon)

Directions:

1. Set the oven at 320 degrees.

2. Cut the banana loaf into thick slices before cutting each slice into halves to form small squares.

3. Spread butter on each slice, then arrange in the oven dish. Pour the blueberries (1 cup) on top of the banana loaf pieces, making sure they are evenly covered. Set aside.

4. Meanwhile, place the coconut cream in a large jug. Add the eggs, vanilla essence, honey, and ½ of the cinnamon. Use an immersion blender to process the ingredients until well-blended and smooth.

5. Add the coconut cream mixture on top of the blueberry-topped banana bread pieces. Use a spatula to spread the mixture evenly. Sprinkle the rest of the cinnamon on the surface, then let sit for about ten minutes.

6. After ten minutes, place in the oven to bake until the bread is light golden brown on top or for about forty minutes.

7. Allow to cool before slicing. Top with yogurt and extra berries.

8. Serve and enjoy.

Easy Apple Crumble

Ingredients:

- Water (1 tablespoon)

- Honey (1 tablespoon)

- Egg (1 piece)

- Cream, cultured, raw/yogurt, plain, nonfat (1 dollop)

- Apples (8 pieces)

- Almond flour (1 cup)

- Vanilla essence (1 teaspoon)

- Almond cookies, crumbled (1 ½ cups)

Directions:

1. Set the oven at 300 degrees.

2. Meanwhile, peel the apples before coring and slicing into thick chunks.

3. Place the apple chunks in a pot. Add water (1 tablespoon) and heat on medium-low. Stew the apples un-

til softened.

4. Once the apples are done, transfer onto a strainer. Once drained, place at the bottom of an oven dish (glass). Set aside.

5. Place the egg in a small bowl. Add honey and vanilla essence. Whisk well to combine, then set aside.

6. Place the almond flour and crumbled almond cookies in a large bowl. Mix well, then pour in the egg mixture. Use a spoon to fold the wet mixture into the dry mixture.

7. Top the stewed apples with the crumble mixture, making sure the apples are evenly covered. Place in the oven to bake for about fifteen to twenty minutes.

8. Once done, remove from the oven and top with yogurt or cream.

9. Slice, serve and enjoy.

Carrot Cupcakes

Ingredients:

- Carrots, grated finely (3 pieces)

- Bicarb (1 teaspoon)

- Coconut flour, organic (1/2 cup)

- Vanilla extract (2 tablespoons)

- Cinnamon (1/2 teaspoon)

- Honey, raw, organic (3/4 cup)

- Dates, pitted, pre-soaked (10 pieces)

- Almond flour, blanched, organic (1 cup)

- Salt (1/2 teaspoon)

- Eggs, free range, organic (10 pieces)

- Coconut oil, melted (2 tablespoons)

Frosting:

- Yogurt, dripped (2 cups)

- Lemon juice, freshly squeezed (2 tablespoons)

- Butter, organic, cultured, warmed to room temp. (100 grams)

- Honey, raw (6 tablespoons)

Directions:

1. Set the oven at 350 degrees to preheat.

2. Grate the carrots into finely shredded pieces, then place in a medium bowl. Add the honey on top of the carrots. Toss to combine before placing in the refrigerator to chill for about twenty minutes.

3. Meanwhile, fill a large bowl with boiling water. Add the dates and allow to sit for about twenty minutes or until softened.

4. Place the eggs in the food processor. Add the dates, honey, yogurt, butter/coconut oil, vanilla extract, and carrot mixture. Process until the mixture is well-blended and has a runny consistency.

5. Add the almond flour, coconut flour, salt, bicarb, and cinnamon. Process again until the mixture is well-combined and thickened.

6. Transfer the prepared batter into a cake tin lined with parchment paper. Spread evenly with a spatula, then place in the oven. Bake for about fifty minutes or until set.

7. Serve and enjoy.

Tasty Pumpkin Bread

Ingredients:

- Almond flour (2 ½ cups)

- Duck fat/coconut oil (1 tablespoon)

- Pumpkin, cooked by boiling (1 ½ cups)

- Eggs (3 pieces)

Directions:

1. Set the oven at 300 degrees to preheat.

2. Place all ingredients in a large bowl. Use a hand mixer to blend all ingredients until just combined, not over-mixed.

3. Meanwhile, use parchment paper to line a bread tin. Pour in the mixture, spread evenly at the bottom of the bread tin, and bake in the oven for about an hour.

4. Once done, take out of the oven immediately to avoid over-burning the loaf. Let cool for ten minutes.

5. Slice and serve.

Delicious Banana Bread

Ingredients:

- Yogurt, plain, nonfat (4 tablespoons)

- Bicarbonate of soda, pure (1 teaspoon)

- Eggs, free range, organic (3 pieces)

- Bananas, ripe, mashed (2 pieces)

- Vanilla essence (1 teaspoon)

- Almond flour, blanched, organic (2 ½ cups)

- Lemon juice (1 tablespoon)

- Honey, raw (2 tablespoons)

- Butter, softened/coconut oil, melted (1 tablespoon)

Directions:

1. Set the oven at 300 degrees to preheat. Meanwhile, use parchment paper to line a bread tin.

2. Place the eggs in a medium bowl. Add the honey,

ghee/butter, and vanilla essence, then whisk well to combine. Set aside.

3. Place the mashed bananas in another large bowl. Add the almond flour as well as the egg mixture. Gently fold in until all ingredients are well-blended.

4. Add the yogurt, lemon juice, and bicarbonate of soda on top of the entire mixture. Use a mixer to blend, then pour into the lined bread tin.

5. Place in the oven to bake for about fifty to fifty-five minutes or until set. Let cool before slicing.

6. Serve and enjoy.

Thank You

As we reach the end of this book, I want to say thanks for reading this book.

I want to get this information out to as many people as possible. If you found this book helpful, I would greatly appreciate you leaving me a review on Amazon. This helps others find the book as well.

Disclaimer

This document is geared towards providing exact and reliable information in regards to the topic and issue covered. The publication is sold on the idea that the publisher is not required to render an accounting, officially permitted, or otherwise, qualified services. If advice is necessary, legal, financial, medical or professional, a practiced individual in the profession should be ordered.

This information is not presented by a financial or medical practitioner and is for entertainment, educational and informational purposes only. The content is not intended as a substitute for professional medical advice, diagnosis, or treatment. Always seek the advice of your physician or other qualified health care provider with any questions you may have regarding a medical condition. Never disregard professional medical advice or delay in seeking it because of something you have read.

The information provided herein is stated to be truthful and consistent, in that any liability, in terms of inattention or otherwise, by any usage or abuse of any policies, processes, or directions contained within is the solitary and utter responsibility of the recipient reader. Under no circumstances will any legal responsibility or blame be held against the

DISCLAIMER

publisher for any reparation, damages, or monetary loss due to the information herein, either directly or indirectly.

Last Updated: 23.May.2017